Making a
difference

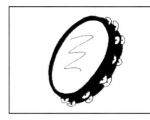 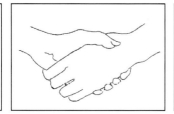 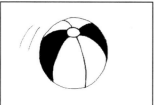

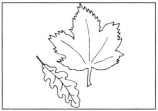  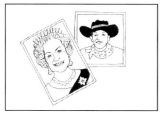

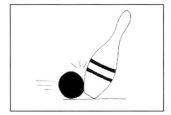 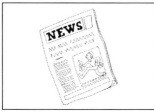 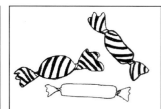

The authors

Aimee Spector and Lene Thorgrimsen were employed as research workers on the Cognitive Stimulation Therapy project at University College London (UCL), which ran from 1997 to 2002. Aimee completed her PhD, based on the project, in 2001 and her Doctorate in Clinical Psychology, also at UCL, in 2004. She is now an Honorary Lecturer at UCL and works as a clinical psychologist in the NHS. Lene completed her PhD, also on the project, in 2003, and is training as a clinical psychologist in Scotland.

Martin Orrell and Bob Woods established and supervised the project. Martin is Professor of Ageing & Mental Health at UCL, and works clinically as an old age psychiatrist in Essex. He is Director of the London Centre for Dementia Care. Bob has worked as a clinical psychologist with people with dementia for 30 years, and was a pioneer of cognitive stimulation approaches such as reality orientation. He is now Professor of Clinical Psychology of Older People at the University of Wales Bangor, and co-director of the Dementia Services Development Centre Wales.

Acknowledgements

The input of Lindsay Royan, Steve Davies, Harry Cayton (on behalf of the Alzheimer's Society), Martin Knapp and the late Margaret Butterworth is gratefully acknowledged. Funding for the project came from the North Thames and London Region NHS Executives, the BHB NHS Trust and the PPP Healthcare Trust.

Making a difference

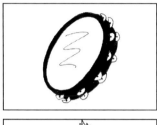 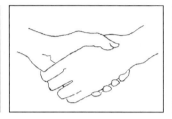 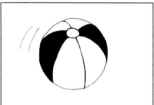

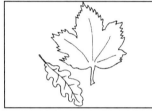 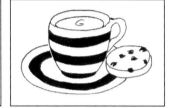 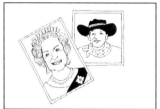

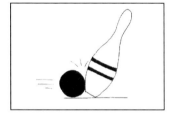 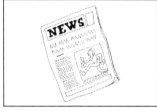 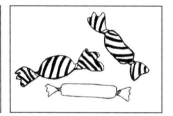

An evidence-based group programme to offer cognitive stimulation therapy (CST) to people with dementia

The manual for group leaders

Aimee Spector, Lene Thorgrimsen
Bob Woods, Martin Orrell

Published by
The Journal for Dementia Care

Making a difference
An evidence-based group programme to offer cognitive stimulation
therapy (CST) to people with dementia – The manual for group leaders

First published in 2006
Reprinted 2007, 2009 (twice), 2010, 2012 (twice), 2013, 2014, 2015, 2016 (twice), 2017

Hawker Publications, Culvert House, Culvert Road, London SW11 5DH
Tel: 020 7720 2108
Fax: 020 7498 3023
Website: www.careinfo.org

© 2006 Department of Mental Health Sciences,
University College London and Dementia Services Development
Centre Wales, University of Wales Bangor

Printed and bound in Great Britain by DG3 Ltd, London

British Library Cataloguing in Publication Data
A catalogue record for this book is available from the British Library
ISBN 9781874 790785

Illustrations by Eve Morris
Book design and layout by Andy Jackson

The North American edition of this manual has been published as
Our Time by Freiberg Press Inc, 2005.

Also published by Hawker Publications:

And still the music plays By Graham Stokes (2008 ISBN 9781874 790884)

Care to communicate – Helping the older person with dementia Jennie Powell (2000 ISBN 9781874 790488)

Chocolate rain By Sarah Zoutewelle-Morris (2011 ISBN 9781874 790969)

Dementia and sexuality By Elaine White (2011 ISBN 9781874 790976)

Dementia Diary By John Killick (2008 ISBN 9781874 790877)

Dementia: Walking not wandering Edited by Mary Marshall and Kate Allan (2006 ISBN 9781874 790686)

Designing homes for people with dementia By Damian Utton (2007 ISBN 9781874 790280)

Food, glorious food – Perspectives on food and dementia. Edited by Mary Marshall (2000 ISBN 9781874 790716)

Making a Difference 2 - with DVD (maintaining CST sessions)
By Elisa Aguirre, Aimée Spector, Amy Streater, Juanita Hoe, Bob Woods and Martin Orrell (2012 ISBN 9781874 790990)

Making a difference 3 : Individual Cognitive Stimulation Therapy : A manual for carers, vol 3
By Lauren Yates, Martin Orrell, Phuong Leung, Aimee Spector, Bob Woods, Vasiliki Orgeta

Time for Dementia – A collection of writings on the meanings of time and dementia
Edited by Jane Gilliard and Mary Marshall. Illustrated by James McKillop (2011 ISBN 9781874 790921)

Watching the leaves dance By Graham Stokes (2016 ISBN 9781874 790402)

Making a difference | Contents

| # Welcome

Over many years of working with staff in hospital wards, residential and nursing homes and day care centres, I have met many nurses and care workers who would like to make a difference. They want to improve the quality of life of the people with dementia they are working with. They would like to reduce the long periods of inactivity which, sadly, are too common a feature of many care centres. They would like to engage those people with dementia who seem to have withdrawn and become apathetic. They would like to get to know the people they are caring for as people, not just as a list of care needs.

How can this be done? It's not easy, of course, to make a real, lasting difference in dementia care. However, I have no doubt that nurses and care workers who become involved in offering the programme described in this manual will take a small but important step to achieving these goals.

It's simple and straightforward
Staff don't need to have special qualifications or attend expensive training courses, and no special equipment is required. All that's needed is for two staff to meet with a small group of people with dementia, in a quiet room, for 45 minutes, twice a week for seven weeks. One of the 'staff' could be a volunteer worker. However, all staff involved must be prepared to follow the key principles of the approach (described on page 7-8), which are the essence of good dementia care.

It's effective
The programme, as described here, was devised from the existing research literature on what is effective in dementia care. It was then evaluated in a large-scale research project (Spector et al 2003). Over 200 people with dementia in care homes and day care centres took part, and were allocated randomly to attend the programme or to receive usual care. Those attending the groups reported increased quality of life compared to those receiving usual care. They actually improved on tests of memory and other abilities, and the conclusion was that the programme was just as effective as the drugs that have been developed to help people with dementia. For the first time, nurses and care workers can be certain of making a real difference to people with dementia, by following this simple programme.

It's enjoyable
Just as important, these groups can be great fun and enjoyable – for people with dementia and for staff. It's great to be able to relax and laugh alongside people with dementia, to see the funny side of a situation together, to see beyond the dementia and to see the real human being. It can be hard work sometimes, of course – every group has its ups and downs – but the experience so far has been that it's a very rewarding programme to be involved in. I hope that's your experience too.

Bob Woods
Professor of Clinical Psychology of Older People
University of Wales, Bangor

Spector A, Thorgrimsen L, Woods B, Royan L, Davies S, Butterworth M, Orrel M (2003) Efficacy of an evidence-based cognitive stimulation therapy programme for people with dementia: randomised controlled trial. British Journal of Psychiatry, 183 248-254.

Key principles

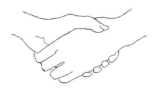

This manual describes a specific programme of group activity and stimulation suitable for use with many people with dementia. Everyone who leads these groups needs to understand, and be ready to put into practice, the following principles of person-centred care. If leaders do not follow these principles there is a real risk that group members will feel patronised, put down or even threatened, with a negative impact on quality of life. This section is not optional!

Person centred

We need to see the person first and foremost, rather than focusing on the dementia and the associated impairments. Each person is unique, with a lifetime of experiences that have shaped their personality and attitudes, leading to a variety of skills, interests, preferences and abilities. Ask yourself about the person's strengths, rather than concentrating on their areas of difficulty. Also, an activity that is appropriate and enjoyable for one person may be disliked intensely by another.

Respect

We need to show respect for the person, and never make them feel small or do anything to expose their difficulties in the group. Help the person to retain their dignity. People with dementia come from all types of cultural and religious backgrounds; show respect by getting to know what is important to each individual, and value the diversity of views, opinions and beliefs within a group. Allow people to be different.

Involvement

If during the group, you find yourself doing most of the talking, or talking 'at' the group, stop! Think about how you can get everyone involved, and offer choices of activities that will interest and engage your particular group. Encourage group members to address their contributions to each other, rather than everything being channelled through the group leader. Remember the group belongs to its members, not to the staff.

Inclusion

Watch out for individuals who appear isolated within the group. If this is due to hearing or vision problems, make arrangements for a leader to sit next to them to ensure they can join in, and make sure the person has their glasses or hearing aid, as appropriate. If the person is a little shy, encourage a more socially active group member to engage with them. If one person in the group has different views or opinions from all the other members, ensure they are not rejected or put down. Encourage an atmosphere where everyone's contribution is valued and respected, and diversity of views is welcomed.

Choice

This group programme is not prescriptive. It is fairly detailed simply to make life easier for group leaders, who will often have many other things on their minds apart from the group. Group members should always be offered choices and alternative activities and approaches found if those offered here do not suit the needs and abilities of your particular group. Offering choices allows group members to become involved in making the group their own – selecting a name for the group, choosing music to use and so on. It goes without saying that no one should be forced to participate in any particular activity. Those who are a little reluctant are more likely to be influenced by seeing others enjoying themselves than by being coerced. For each session, we have suggested a choice of activities (described as Level A and Level B), often geared to groups at different levels of ability. Usually Level B activities are less demanding on the person's memory and other cognitive skills. Choose which seems most appropriate for your group, or mix activities from the two levels, or add your own ideas. There is space throughout this manual to note activities you have tried for each session, so that next time around they can be among the choices open to you.

Fun

Sometimes group members will say "This is like being back in school". If they mean by this that they are being made to work hard in a strict and serious atmosphere, something is going wrong. The groups should provide a learning atmosphere which is fun and enjoyable with a group of friends. Yes, members' brains should be stimulated, but so should their laughter muscles! If members make comments about 'school', ask them what they liked and disliked about school, and reflect on whether the group leaders are taking on the role of 'teacher' too readily. Avoid using equipment that is, or looks like it is, intended for children (apart from when reminiscing about childhood). Group members are adults and we must ensure that nothing we do treats them like children.

Opinions rather than facts

In group sessions, we need to focus on people's strengths. If we focus on 'facts' too much, there is the risk that people will often be wrong. If we ask people for their opinions, then they may be amusing, sad, unusual, controversial or puzzling, but they cannot be wrong. Everyone in the group is entitled to their own opinion, of course. So, rather than say "Where did you go on holiday when you were a child?" (a memory question), ask "What's your favourite place to go on holiday?" or "Where would you advise a young family to go on holiday?". Rather than ask "Who is the Prime Minister?", ask "What do you think of politicians?" or "Who has been the best leader of the country?", in the latter case giving a range of names, backed up by photographs. The group should never feel like a memory test. Avoid questions beginning "Who can remember…?".

Using reminiscence

Using past memories is an excellent way of tapping into a strength many people with dementia have: the ability to recall experiences from much earlier in their lives. For many, it is also an enjoyable activity. Remember, though, that some people with dementia may have unhappy (even traumatic) memories of their earlier life, and some sensitivity is needed not to push members into exposing painful memories in the group setting. If a raw nerve is touched upon accidentally, take time with the person (on a one-to-one basis) to enable them to talk further, if they wish, or to regain their composure. The better you know the backgrounds and life stories of group members, the less likely this is to occur, but unforeseeable areas of difficulty may still emerge.

Using the senses – multi-sensory stimulation

There will be differences between members in their preferred sense (that is, the sense which is most effective and powerful for the individual). Try to ensure that you have a variety of sensory stimuli, with a mix of activities involving vision, touch, hearing, taste and smell. Often it is a combination that is most effective. For example, a scented candle offers a pleasant smell, the sight of the flame flickering and the feel of the heat being radiated. Think about the way you communicate, making sure that you use non-verbal means of communication as well as verbal. Your facial expression, tone of voice, posture and gestures will speak volumes.

Always have something to look at, touch or feel

The group programme presented here always offers a focus for members. Words in a discussion may soon be lost when memory is limited; having an object, a photograph or picture there keeps members' attention on the activity and encourages a group focus.

Maximising potential

Be careful not to assume that a person with dementia is unable to contribute or carry out an activity simply because they were not able to yesterday or last week. People with dementia often function at less than their full potential, perhaps due to lack of stimulation or opportunity. There is evidence that, with the right encouragement, people with dementia can learn. This involves giving the person time, being careful not to overload or overwhelm them with information, and providing just enough prompts to enable the person to carry out the activity themselves. This will increase exposure to success, which also will aid learning and enjoyment. People with dementia are likely to achieve their potential by doing, rather than by sitting passively and watching.

Building and strengthening relationships

The group sessions will help members get to know each other better, and can strengthen relationships between the members and leaders – especially if the leaders ensure they do not become 'teacher', but assist members, join in, have fun and don't present themselves as all-knowing experts. Person-centred care means allowing yourself to be a person, an ordinary human being, in person-to-person relationships with people with dementia. That's not easy, but in a small group, away from some of the care-giving pressures, it's possible and very worthwhile.

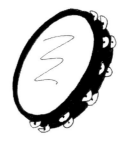

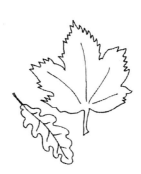

Getting started

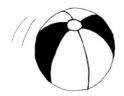

How many members?
We recommend a maximum of five or six people.

How many leaders?
It's difficult to run a group on your own. We suggest you need two regular leaders who can be at every session. Leaders can be staff or volunteers; they need to understand and follow the key principles described previously.

Who to include?
It's worth taking time to think about who you will invite to the group. First of all identify potential members who have some degree of dementia or memory problems and some ability to communicate. Then ask these key questions:

- Does the person have a severe hearing impairment (even with any aid)?

- Does the person have a severe visual impairment (even with glasses)?

- Is the person too agitated to remain in the group?

- Does the person have severe physical health problems that will affect the person's ability to attend the groups?

If the answer to any of these questions is 'yes', the person is unlikely to benefit from a group programme, and will need other forms of support and help.

Before finalising group membership consider the gender balance of the group, in relation to individual preferences: some men enjoy being the only male in a group, but others hate it.

Try not to have too big a range of ability in the group, as some members become

Your notes

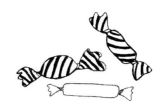

frustrated with those who are struggling to keep up. Obviously, if there are people who you know do not get on with each other, it may be best not to invite them to the same group.

Time

The programme is designed to take place over two sessions per week, each of 45 minutes, but you need to allow an hour to give time for gathering members together and for a few minutes of reflection at the end.

Place

You will need to find a separate, comfortable room; it should be quiet and definitely not a thoroughfare. It should be equipped with a whiteboard.

Equipment

Before starting, if the unit does not already have them, consider purchasing the following items (* indicates these are essential – others are open to improvisation):

- whiteboard and pens*

- soft ball*

- tape-recorder and/or CD player*

- song books*

- tapes and/or CDs of music enjoyed by group members*

- skittles/indoor bowls/boules

- sound effects tapes

- old-fashioned toys (for example, a spinning top, jacks, hoopla) – these may be borrowed from a reminiscence collection or from someone's attic!

Your notes

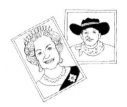

- selection of grocery replicas (available from toyshops)

- photographs of local scenes – past and present, including old postcards of the area

- large map of the country

- photographs of famous faces

- Polaroid camera or digital camera and printer

- trivia quiz books

- dominoes, playing cards, bingo.

For some sessions multiple copies of materials are required. Access to a colour photocopier and to a laminator can help in preparing these.

A number of useful resources, including some of those used in this programme, are available from:

Speechmark Publishers Ltd.
Telford Road
Bicester
Oxfordshire OX26 4LQ
Tel: 01869 244644

www.speechmark.net

Your notes

Monitoring progress

It is important to keep a session by session record of each member's response to and involvement in the sessions to enable you to adapt and plan the programme for future sessions. Photocopy this page to keep a record of the whole group programme.

Session number.........

For each member, rate their interest, communication, enjoyment and mood shown in today's session with a number from 1 to 5 as follows (use 2s and 4s to reflect ratings in between the descriptions given):

Names of members	Attended? Yes/No	Interest	Communication	Enjoyment	Mood
1.					
2.					
3.					
4.					
5.					
6.					

Interest:
- 1 = No interest
- 3 = Shows some interest
- 5 = Shows great interest

Communication:
- 1 = Little or no communication
- 3 = Some response
- 5 = Communicates well

Enjoyment:
- 1 = Does not show enjoyment of the session today
- 3 = Shows some enjoyment
- 5 = Enjoys the session greatly

Mood:
- 1 = In low mood today, appears depressed or anxious
- 3 = Some signs of good mood
- 5 = Appears happy and relaxed today

Activities used today:

Comments:

This page may be photocopied

Physical games

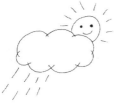

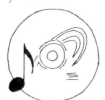

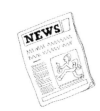

Introductions (10 minutes)

Welcome all members individually to the group, by name.

Involve everyone in a discussion about giving the group a name. Generate two or three possible names, write them on the whiteboard, and have a vote. Write the winning name prominently on the board.

As a group, select a 'theme song' for the group, then sing it together (use song book or music tape). Ask for a group member to act as song leader.

Discuss day, month, year, season, weather, time, name and address of the centre (use whiteboard).

Discuss something currently in the news (use newspapers or photographs).

Offer refreshments.

Your ideas

Main activity (25 minutes)

Level A
Throw a soft ball around, asking people to say something about themselves as they catch the ball, for example, their name, where they come from, their former occupation, favourite food or colour.

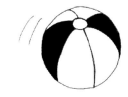

Level B
Play a physical game, such as skittles or indoor bowls or boules, which involves teamwork. This should be a relaxed activity incorporating movement, touch and score calculations.

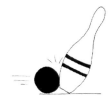

Finally… (10 minutes)

Thank everyone individually for attending and contributing.

Sing theme song again.

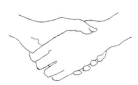

Remind everyone of the time and content of the next session.

Say farewells.

Your ideas

Sounds

Introductions (10 minutes)

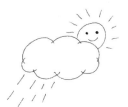

Welcome all members individually to the group, by name.

Draw attention to the name of the group (on the whiteboard). Remind everyone of the activity in the last session.

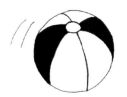

Play soft-ball game for a few minutes. When throwing the ball, people may either state their own name, or, for the more able, the name of the person to whom they are throwing the ball. Vary this by asking people to say their favourite food, colour, sport, town, country, film star, singer and so on).

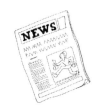

Sing together the group's 'theme song', led by song leader (use song book or tape).

Discuss day, month, year, season, time, name and address of the centre (use whiteboard).

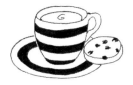

Discuss opinions of recent events in the centre, for example, recent meals or the weather yesterday and today. Discuss something currently in the news (use newspapers or photographs).

Offer refreshments.

Your ideas

Main activity (25 minutes)

Level A

Play sound effects tapes that include different categories, such as 'indoor sounds' and 'outdoor sounds' (for example, animal noises) and invite members to match the sounds with pictures. This gives people both visual and auditory stimulation, making the task easier. Alternatively, play selected tracks from a compilation music CD from the appropriate era and invite members to name the song or singer. If necessary, provide a choice of two or three names on the whiteboard as members listen to the song.

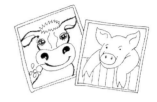

Level B

Give percussion instruments (including things like spoons, combs with paper and so on) to each person in the group, and use them to play along to familiar music, such as popular 1940s music.

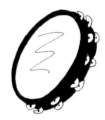

Finally... (10 minutes)

Summarise today's discussion and seek feedback about the session. Thank everyone individually for attending and contributing.

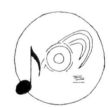

Sing theme song again.

Remind everyone of the time and content of the next session.

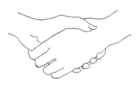

Say farewells.

Your ideas

Childhood

Introductions (10 minutes)

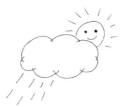

Welcome all members individually to the group, by name.

Draw attention to the name of the group (on the whiteboard). Remind everyone of the activity in the last session.

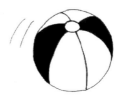

Play soft-ball game for a few minutes. As in Session 2, use a variety of categories for members to call out when catching the ball.

Sing together the group's 'theme song', led by song leader (use song book or tape).

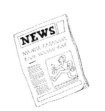

Discuss day, month, year, season, time, name and address of the centre (use whiteboard).

Discuss opinions of recent events in the centre, for example, recent meals or the weather yesterday and today. Discuss something currently in the news (use newspapers or photographs).

Offer refreshments.

Your ideas

Main activity (25 minutes)

Level A

Ask members to fill out a printed sheet with their name, father's name, mother's name, schools attended and so on to form the first page of a memory diary (see record sheet on page 21). Invite people to make a plan or drawing of their childhood bedroom, or even create a reconstruction of it on a board.

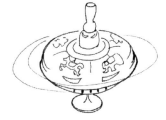

Level B

Ask members to demonstrate the use of old-fashioned childhood toys, for example, a spinning top, jacks and hoopla. Talk about childhood sweets: liquorice, pear drops, aniseed balls, gobstoppers, bullseyes, barley sugar, treacle toffee, sherbet fountains. Bring a selection to try and enjoy!

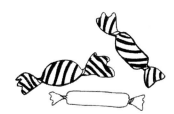

Finally... (10 minutes)

Summarise today's discussion and seek feedback about the session. Thank everyone individually for attending and contributing.

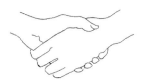

Sing theme song again.

Remind everyone of the time and content of the next session.

Say farewells.

Your ideas

My childhood

Name ....

I was born on ....

at ....

My mother was called ....

My father was called ....

I had .... brothers and .... sisters.

Their names were ....

....

We lived at ....

Other important people in my family were ....

....

I went to school at ....

and ....

My best subjects were ....

My worst subjects were ....

My best friends at school were ....

I left school aged ....

My first job was ....

Food

Introductions (10 minutes)

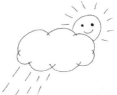

Welcome all members individually to the group, by name.

Draw attention to the name of the group (on the whiteboard). Remind everyone of the activity in the last session.

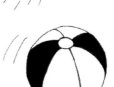

Play soft-ball game for a few minutes. As in Session 2 use a variety of categories for members to call out when catching the ball.

Sing together the group's 'theme song' led by song leader (use song book or tape).

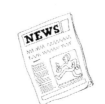

Discuss day, month, year, season, time, name and address of the centre (use whiteboard).

Discuss opinions of recent events in the centre, for example, recent meals or the weather yesterday and today. Discuss something currently in the news (use newspapers or photographs).

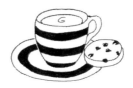

Offer refreshments.

Your ideas

Main activity (25 minutes)

Level A
Using real groceries or miniature grocery replicas that have been priced, give people a budget and a scenario to plan, for example, a dinner for four.

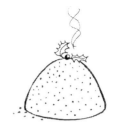

Categorise the groceries into foods for different mealtimes, special occasions, savoury/sweet.

Level B
Taste foods which act as memory triggers or have personal meaning, for example, cream soda, ginger beer, bread pudding, Bovril.

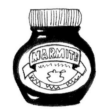

Brainstorm food categories on the whiteboard, such as soups, meats, puddings, fish, vegetables. List as many as possible in each category.

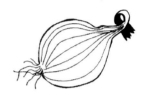

Complete names of food items, for example, Yorkshire ..., Bakewell ... and self-raising ....

Ask people to name foods beginning with a particular letter.

Finally... (10 minutes)

Summarise today's discussion and seek feedback about the session. Thank everyone individually for attending and contributing.

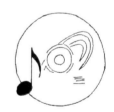

Sing theme song again.

Remind everyone of the time and content of the next session.

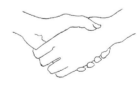

Say farewells.

> Your ideas

Current affairs

Introductions (10 minutes)

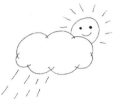

Welcome all members individually to the group, by name.

Draw attention to the name of the group (on the whiteboard). Remind everyone of the activity in the last session.

Play soft-ball game for a few minutes. As in Session 2 use a variety of categories for members to call out when catching the ball.

Sing together the group's 'theme song', led by song leader (use song book or tape).

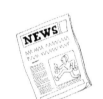

Discuss day, month, year, season, time, name and address of the centre (use whiteboard).

Discuss opinions of recent events in the centre, for example, recent meals or the weather yesterday and today. Discuss something currently in the news (use newspapers or photographs).

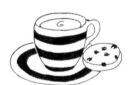

Offer refreshments.

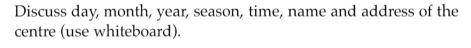

Your ideas

Main activity (25 minutes)

Level A
Discuss issues from a selection of recent national and local newspapers and picture magazines. Have multiple copies of interesting articles (laminated if possible) so everyone has the same piece to look at.

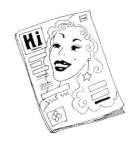

Level B
Use questions on cue cards to stimulate conversation on news, views, attitudes, dreams and aspirations. Some examples of opening questions might be:

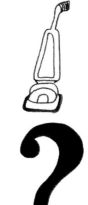

- Should men and women have different roles? Should men do the cooking, cleaning and laundry?
- What do you think of today's fashion?
- What do you think of gay weddings?
- What's your opinion of the royal family? Would we be better off without them?
- What's your favourite charity?
- Who in the world do you admire most?
- Where is your favourite place in the world?
- Are mobile phones a good thing? (Demonstrate if necessary.)
- Should there be a retirement age for everyone? What should it be?
- Is it too easy now to get a divorce?

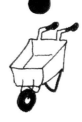

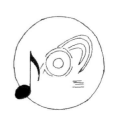

Finally… (10 minutes)

Summarise today's discussion and seek feedback about the session. Thank everyone individually for attending and contributing.

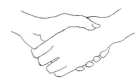

Sing theme song again.

Remind everyone of the time and content of the next session.

Say farewells.

Your ideas

SESSION SIX | **Faces/scenes**

Introductions (10 minutes)

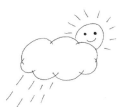

Welcome all members individually to the group, by name.

Draw attention to the name of the group (on the whiteboard). Remind everyone of the activity in the last session.

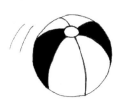

Play soft-ball game for a few minutes. As in Session 2 use a variety of categories for members to call out when catching the ball.

Sing together the group's 'theme song' led by song leader (use song book or tape).

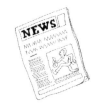

Discuss day, month, year, season, time, name and address of the centre (use whiteboard).

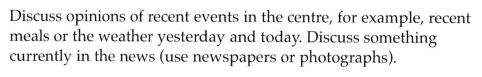

Discuss opinions of recent events in the centre, for example, recent meals or the weather yesterday and today. Discuss something currently in the news (use newspapers or photographs).

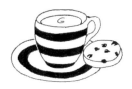

Offer refreshments.

Your ideas

Main activity (25 minutes)

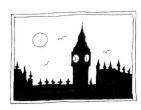

Level A
Prepare multiple copies of laminated photographs of famous faces or of local scenes (for example, from old postcards) so that everyone can look at the same picture. Give people one or more cards and ask them to identify the person or scene. Allow discussion of people's memories of these people or places to flow.

Level B
Use the same types of prepared cards as in Level A, but ask for people's opinions, such as:

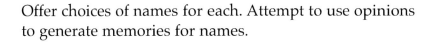
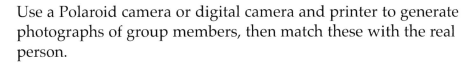

• Who is the most attractive?
• Who is the oldest, or youngest?
• What do they have in common?
• How are they different?

Offer choices of names for each. Attempt to use opinions to generate memories for names.

Use a Polaroid camera or digital camera and printer to generate photographs of group members, then match these with the real person.

Finally… (10 minutes)

Summarise today's discussion and seek feedback about the session. Thank everyone individually for attending and contributing.

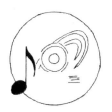

Sing theme song again.

Remind everyone of the time and content of the next session.

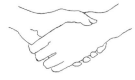

Say farewells.

Your ideas

| # Word association

Introductions (10 minutes)

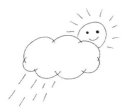

Welcome all members individually to the group, by name.

Draw attention to the name of the group (on the whiteboard). Remind everyone of the activity in the last session.

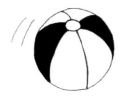

Play soft-ball game for a few minutes. As in Session 2 use a variety of categories for members to call out when catching the ball.

Sing together the group's 'theme song', led by song leader (use song book or tape).

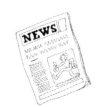

Discuss day, month, year, season, time, name and address of the centre (use whiteboard).

Discuss opinions of recent events in the centre, for example, recent meals or the weather yesterday and today. Discuss something currently in the news (use newspapers or photographs).

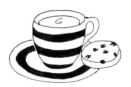

Offer refreshments.

Your ideas

Main activity (25 minutes)

Level A
Ask group members to supply the missing word in a number of phrases. These could be about quantities (a cup of ...), famous couples (Laurel and ...), famous places (Westminster ...) or proverbs (A stitch in time ...). See the lists below for more examples.

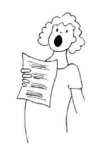

Level B
Present the first few words of a song (for example, 'We'll meet again ...') and ask the group to sing a few lines.

Finally... (10 minutes)

Summarise today's discussion and seek feedback about the session. Thank everyone individually for attending and contributing.

Sing theme song again.

Remind everyone of the time and content of the next session.

Say farewells.

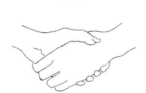

Missing words: some examples

Quantities
cup of . . . . tea, coffee
loaf of . . . . bread
slice of . . . . bread, cake, ham, life
jug of . . . . water, milk, beer
pint of . . . . milk, beer
gallon of. . . . . petrol
reel of . . . . cotton
ball of . . . . wool
pair of . . . . shoes, trousers, glasses
bucket of . . . . water, sand

Couples
Laurel and . . . . Hardy
Morecambe and . . . . Wise
Marks and . . . . Spencer
Little and . . . . Large
Crosse and . . . . Blackwell

Places
Westminster . . . . Abbey
Buckingham . . . . Palace
Windsor . . . . Castle
Trafalgar . . . . Square
Piccadilly . . . . Circus
Nelson's . . . . Column
Waterloo . . . . Bridge, station
Canterbury . . . . Cathedral
Charing . . . . Cross
New . . . . -castle
Coronation. . . . . Street
Isle of . . . . Wight

Proverbs
A stitch in time . . . . saves nine.
Make hay while . . . . the sun shines.
A watched kettle never . . . . boils.
The grass is always greener . . . . . . on the other side.
A bird in the hand is worth . . . . two in the bush.
Strike while the iron is . . . . hot.

Being creative

Introductions (10 minutes)

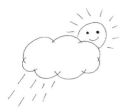

Welcome all members individually to the group, by name.

Draw attention to the name of the group (on the whiteboard). Remind everyone of the activity in the last session.

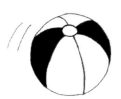

Play soft-ball game for a few minutes. As in Session 2 use a variety of categories for members to call out when catching the ball.

Sing together the group's 'theme song', led by song leader (use song book or tape).

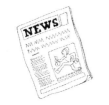

Discuss day, month, year, season, time, name and address of the centre (use whiteboard).

Discuss opinions of recent events in the centre, for example, recent meals or the weather yesterday and today. Discuss something currently in the news (use newspapers or photographs).

Offer refreshments.

Your ideas

Main activity (25 minutes)

Levels A and B

In this session, do a creative activity such as:

- cookery: make an apple crumble or similar dish. Split the activity into separate tasks (greasing the bowl, mixing ingredients, making crumble mixture, peeling and slicing apples) so that everyone can participate.

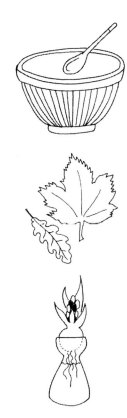

- making a seasonal collage: use natural items (for example, autumn leaves or spring flowers) and pictures to create a collage.

- Clay modelling: make animals or sculptures out of clay.

- Gardening: plant bulbs or seeds and check their progress in future weeks.

Finally… (10 minutes)

Summarise the discussion and seek feedback about the session. Thank everyone individually for attending and contributing.

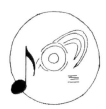

Sing theme song again.

Remind everyone of the time and content of the next session.

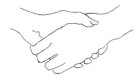

Say farewells.

Your ideas

SESSION NINE | **Categorising objects**

Introductions (10 minutes)

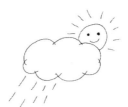

Welcome all members individually to the group, by name.

Draw attention to the name of the group (on the whiteboard). Remind everyone of the activity in the last session.

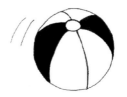

Play soft-ball game for a few minutes. As in Session 2 use a variety of categories for members to call out when catching the ball.

Sing together the group's 'theme song', led by song leader (use song book or tape).

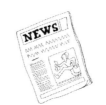

Discuss day, month, year, season, time, name and address of the centre (use whiteboard).

Discuss opinions of recent events in the centre, for example, recent meals or the weather yesterday and today. Discuss something currently in the news (use newspapers or photographs).

Offer refreshments.

Your ideas

Making a difference

Main activity (25 minutes)

Level A

Ask people to think of words beginning with a certain letter (say 'A') in a particular category (say 'boys' names'). Write letters and categories on separate cards and use the cards to prompt the game. Alternatively, simply write the category on the board and invite people to think of as many examples as possible.

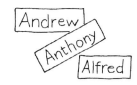

Level B

Place 20 or so objects or coloured pictures of objects on a table. Ask people to group the objects in different ways, for example, by use, colour or initial letter. This can be done as an 'odd one out' game, that is, by asking which of three objects is the odd one out.

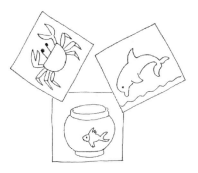

Finally… (10 minutes)

Summarise today's discussion and seek feedback about the session. Thank everyone individually for attending and contributing.

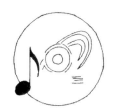

Sing theme song again.

Remind everyone of the time and content of the next session.

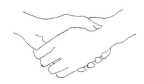

Say farewells.

Categories: some examples

1. countries
2. boys' names
3. girls' names
4. vegetables
5. flowers
6. alcoholic drinks
7. things to do with Christmas
8. famous singers
9. foods
10. towns/cities
11. world leaders (past and present)
12. animals
13. birds
14. films
15. songs
16. things found in the supermarket
17. things found in the kitchen
18. things found in the shed
19. things found in the garden
20. musical instruments
21. fish
22. colours
23. items of clothing
24. means of transport
25. things you fear
26. things you enjoy
27. film stars
28. TV programmes
29. sports
30. counties/states

| **Orientation**

Introductions (10 minutes)

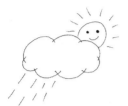

Welcome all members individually to the group, by name.

Draw attention to the name of the group (on the whiteboard). Remind everyone of the activity in the last session.

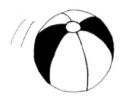

Play soft-ball game for a few minutes. As in Session 2 use a variety of categories for members to call out when catching the ball.

Sing together the group's 'theme song', led by song leader (use song book or tape).

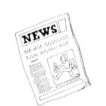

Discuss day, month, year, season, time, name and address of the centre (use whiteboard).

Discuss opinions of recent events in the centre, for example, recent meals or the weather yesterday and today. Discuss something currently in the news (use newspapers or photographs).

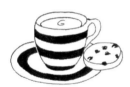

Offer refreshments.

Your ideas

Main activity (25 minutes)

Level A

Depending on where group members come from, construct a map of the UK, the local area or the centre on whiteboard. Fill in the 'map' by asking the group to suggest different places or landmarks, such as a favourite seaside destination (on the UK map), the post office (on the local area map) or the dining room (on a plan of the centre), then draw them in the appropriate position on the map. Some towns/cities have 'then and now' photograph books that document changes during the 20th century – use these to stimulate discussion if most members know the area.

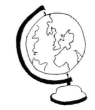

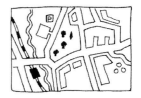

Level B

Mark on a large map where group members originate from. Discuss whether people have moved from area to area, and if so, where from and to. If members have travelled abroad, use a map of the world to identify the different places. Discuss how long journeys take, how far apart places are, transport links and landmarks.

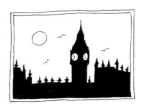

Finally… (10 minutes)

Summarise the discussion and seek feedback about the session. Thank everyone individually for attending and contributing.

Sing theme song again.

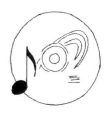

Remind everyone of the time and content of the next session.

Say farewells.

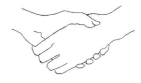

```
Your ideas



```

Using money

Introductions (10 minutes)

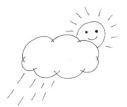

Welcome all members individually to the group, by name.

Draw attention to the name of the group (on the whiteboard). Remind everyone of the activity in the last session.

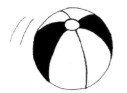

Play soft-ball game for a few minutes. As in Session 2 use a variety of categories for members to call out when catching the ball.

Sing together the group's 'theme song', led by song leader (use song book or tape).

Discuss day, month, year, season, time, name and address of the centre (use whiteboard).

Discuss opinions of recent events in the centre, for example, recent meals or the weather yesterday and today. Discuss something currently in the news (use newspapers or photographs).

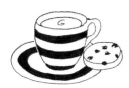

Offer refreshments.

Your ideas

Main activity (25 minutes)

Level A

Prepare laminated cut-outs of common objects from a catalogue (or have actual objects there) with prices marked on the back. Ask people to guess the price of items, add up prices ('How much will the total bill be?'), or match the price tag with the object.

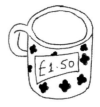

Level B

Show examples of both old and new coins and compare these. Discuss changes in prices and values using questions such as:

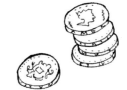

- How much was your first pay packet?
- How much did people used to earn?
- How much did a loaf of bread cost?
- What can you get for £5 now?

Finally... (10 minutes)

Summarise the discussion and seek feedback about the session. Thank everyone individually for attending and contributing.

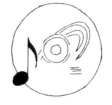

Sing theme song again.

Remind everyone of the time and content of the next session.

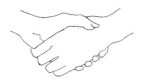

Say farewells.

Your ideas

Number games

Introductions (10 minutes)

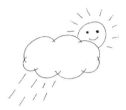

Welcome all members individually to the group, by name.

Draw attention to the name of the group (on the whiteboard). Remind everyone of the activity in the last session.

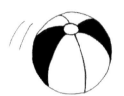

Play soft-ball game for a few minutes. As in Session 2 use a variety of categories for members to call out when catching the ball.

Sing together the group's 'theme song', led by song leader (use song book or tape).

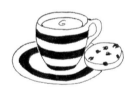

Discuss day, month, year, season, time, name and address of the centre (use whiteboard).

Discuss opinions of recent events in the centre, for example, recent meals or the weather yesterday and today. Discuss something currently in the news (use newspapers or photographs).

Offer refreshments.

Your ideas

Main activity (25 minutes)

Level A
Play games involving the recognition and use of numbers, for example, bingo or dominoes.

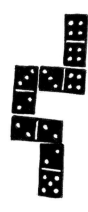

Level B
Play 'snap' with playing cards.

Go around the group, with each person in turn taking the next card off a pack of cards and guessing whether it will be higher or lower than the previous card.

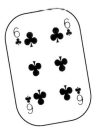

Guess how many items are in a container (for example, pennies in a small jar). Count them out to check whose guess is closest!

Finally… (10 minutes)

Summarise the discussion and seek feedback about the session. Thank everyone individually for attending and contributing.

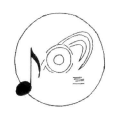

Sing theme song again.

Remind everyone of the time and content of the next session.

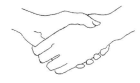

Say farewells.

Your ideas

Word games

Introductions (10 minutes)

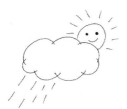

Welcome all members individually to the group, by name.

Draw attention to the name of the group (on the whiteboard). Remind everyone of the activity in the last session.

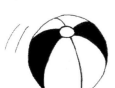

Play soft-ball game for a few minutes. As in Session 2 use a variety of categories for members to call out when catching the ball.

Sing together the group's 'theme song', led by song leader (use song book or tape).

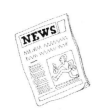

Discuss day, month, year, season, time, name and address of the centre (use whiteboard).

Discuss opinions of recent events in the centre, for example, recent meals or the weather yesterday and today. Discuss something currently in the news (use newspapers or photographs).

Offer refreshments.

Your ideas

Main activity (25 minutes)

Level A
Play a word identification game such as 'hangman' which involves the recognition and use of letters and words. Draw a number of dashes for each letter of a word, and ask the group to guess the letters. Incorrect letters contribute, one by one, to the drawing of a 'hangman' and losing the game. The group is required to guess the word – if needed, give a category clue (for example, type of drink).

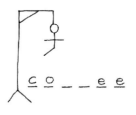

Level B
Prepare a large-size crossword or word search puzzle on A3 paper at a difficulty level geared to the group.

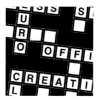

Finally… (10 minutes)

Summarise the discussion and seek feedback about the session. Thank everyone individually for attending and contributing.

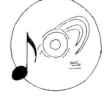

Sing theme song again.

Remind everyone of the time and content of the next session.

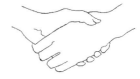

Say farewells.

Your ideas

Team quiz

Introductions (10 minutes)

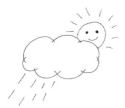

Welcome all members individually to the group, by name.

Draw attention to the name of the group (on the whiteboard). Remind everyone of the activity in the last session.

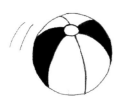

Play soft-ball game for a few minutes. As in Session 2 use a variety of categories for members to call out when catching the ball.

Sing together the group's 'theme song', led by song leader (use song book or tape).

Discuss day, month, year, season, time, name and address of the centre (use whiteboard).

Discuss opinions of recent events in the centre, for example, recent meals or the weather yesterday and today. Discuss something currently in the news (use newspapers or photographs)

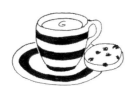

Offer light refreshments, although a special tea is to follow.

Your ideas

Main activity (25 minutes)

Levels A and B
Play team games: divide the group into two teams, ask them to choose a team name and then play trivia quiz, or another game the group have enjoyed previously. Give prizes to everyone in the group.

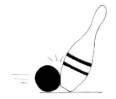

Bring back materials created in previous sessions and display for all to see.

Have a special group tea with cakes, special treats and so on.

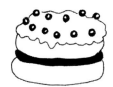

Discuss people's views on the group.

Finally… (10 minutes)

Summarise today's discussion and seek feedback about the overall group experience. Thank everyone individually for attending and contributing.

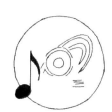

Sing theme song again.

Say farewells.

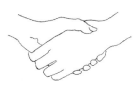

Your ideas

What's next?

Maintenance sessions

We have found that continuing with sessions once a week helps to maintain the improvements in memory that were observed following the initial 14 session programme for at least another four months (Orrell *et al* 2005).

These maintenance sessions followed similar themes, but tried to use different materials wherever possible as it is important that boredom is avoided for both members and leaders.

The structure for each session was similar to that used for the first 14 sessions. As a guide, we list here the specific activities used in the 16 maintenance sessions. These may, of course, be mixed or substituted according to group members' interests and preferences.

1. Childhood: questions from the record sheets were used as prompts for discussion (such as 'Describe your childhood bedroom'). Childhood toys and games were included.
2. Current affairs: duplicate copies of discussion-provoking articles from newspapers were used to generate opinion and debate.
3. Current affairs: as for previous session.
4. Using objects: making a chocolate cake.
5. Number game: bingo.
6. Quiz: involving two teams.
7. Music session: this involved the playing of musical instruments, singing along to old songs and a 'song completion' game where people are given the first few words of a song and are asked to sing the remainder.

8. Physical games: such as hoopla, skittles, boules and football. The group was encouraged to calculate the scores.
9. Categorising objects: 'odd one out' game, with four words written on a sheet of paper and the group asked to guess the 'odd one out' (for example, banana, orange, margarine, pineapple). Naming objects from a particular category beginning with a certain letter (an item of clothing beginning with 'B').
10. Using objects: reminiscence materials and modern objects (such as a mobile phone) were presented and discussed.
11. Useful tips: a book about customs and remedies from the past was used to generate a discussion about useful tips – how to soothe burns, keep milk fresh, and so on.
12. Discussion topics: cards asking discussion-provoking questions were passed around the group ('What is your favourite charity?' or 'How are elderly people treated by society today?').
13. Discussion topics: as for previous session.
14. Discussion about people's opinions of different types of art, generated through the presentation of pictures of art works, ranging from classical to modern.
15. Famous faces: pictures of people from the past used to make comparisons and generate discussion.
16. Word completion: completion of proverbs and 'famous couples'.

Orrell M, Spector A, Thorgrimsen L, Woods R (2005) A pilot study examining the effectiveness of maintenance cognitive stimulation therapy (CST) following CST for people with dementia. *International Journal of Geriatric Psychiatry* 20 446-451.

Other types of group work

There are many other forms of group work that may also be useful with people with dementia and will add to the variety of stimulation and experience. These include creative therapy groups (such as art and music groups), physical exercise sessions, reminiscence groups, aromatherapy, hand massage and so on.

Useful resources for developing new ideas

We recommend the following sources of ideas and information on person-centred care and therapeutic approaches in dementia care:

Journal of Dementia Care
www.careinfo.org/dementiacare
Useful practitioner magazine; also has a range of publications and conferences.

Hawker Publications
Culvert House
Culvert Road
London SW11 5DH
Tel: 020 7720 2108 ext. 206

Signpost
www.signpostjournal.co.uk
Also a practitioner magazine with useful articles and reviews, and announcements of conferences and training events.

Practice Development Unit (MHSOP)
Whitchurch Hospital
Park Road
Cardiff CF14 7BP
Tel: 029 2033 6073

Alzheimer's Society
www.alzheimers.org.uk
Useful website, publications, training materials and courses.

Gordon House
10 Greencoat Place
London SW1P 1PH
Tel: 020 7306 0606

Dementia Services Development Centres (DSDCs)
Links can be found on the DSDC Wales website at www.bangor.ac.uk/dsdc
Publications, courses, training.

Ardudwy, University of Wales, Bangor
Holyhead Road
Bangor
Gwynedd LL57 2PX
Tel: 01248 383719

Bradford Dementia Group
www.brad.ac.uk/health/bdg
Useful publications on person-centred care and many courses and training events.

Bradford Dementia Group
School of Health Studies
University of Bradford
25 Trinity Road
Bradford BD5 0BB
Tel: 01274 235726

Cognitive Stimulation Therapy website
www.cstdementia.com
Developed by the authors of this manual, this site provides updates on the approach, information about training and new resources, as they become available.

Frequently asked questions

Can anything actually be done for people with dementia?

It is quite common for people to feel hopeless when they first think about working with people with dementia. After all, the conditions which cause dementia can have serious consequences, and many will have witnessed people with dementia losing more and more abilities as time goes on. However, there is in fact good evidence that people with dementia can learn, in certain circumstances, and do respond to their environment, and through programmes such as this one can experience an improvement in quality of life. We may not yet be able to reverse the course of dementia, but some of the major difficulties for people with dementia are caused by understimulation, withdrawal, depression and anxiety, and these can be reduced. This can make a real difference to the person and those who care about him/her. We need to look for small, subtle changes that make a difference to the person's life.

What if I've tried activities before but nobody ever seems interested?

If you are working with a group of people who, for whatever reason, have lost motivation, it can be really difficult to get them involved again. We have found it helpful to: describe beforehand what you will be doing; warn people in advance about the group meeting coming up (display an attractive notice in a prominent place advertising the meeting); show some of the interesting materials you plan to use; have the group in a room that is easy for people to get to; and offer good refreshments! It may be necessary to engage some individuals with the materials before bringing them into the group.

What if people shout over each other or don't listen?

It's difficult for any of us if we're in a group or a meeting where everyone is talking at once, and for people with dementia it can be overwhelming. The most important role of group leaders is to make sure this doesn't happen. It is important to arrange the seating so that leaders are sitting next to group members who are hard of hearing or a little anxious. Going round the group, asking each person's opinion in turn is a good strategy for ensuring everyone has the chance to have their say. Gently bring the group back to the topic – using a tangible focus – if the discussion is going off in several different directions at once. Sometimes it may be necessary to break into two smaller groups, with one leader in each, with each subgroup then bringing a summary of its opinions back to the whole group after a few minutes.

Does it need to be the same people each week?

There are benefits of having a 'closed' group, where the same people meet for the 14 sessions. People get to know each other and become familiar with the routine of the group. Leaders get to know the members and can plan activities according to their interests. Obviously, not everyone will be able to attend all sessions, through illness, outside appointments and so on. However, it is important that once the person has joined the group it be given priority so they will derive the maximum benefit from the experience.

What happens if leaders miss some sessions?

Sickness and unavoidable absence always occur, but staff rotas should be geared to ensure the group has consistency of leadership. If one leader is absent, the other can continue, but will need the assistance of another staff member. It is inadvisable to try to lead a group session single-handed unless the number of members is very small (three or less).

What if issues arise that people find upsetting?

The discussion about reminiscence work in the 'Key principles' section (see page 7) deals with this type of situation. People with dementia, like anyone else, become upset from time to time, and leaders have the role of providing support (which may mean giving some space or a quiet chat over a cup of tea) when this occurs. Sometimes a person suddenly becomes upset if they find themselves failing something that was previously second nature to them. As far as possible, the sessions are designed to avoid this experience of failure, but it can occur at times in any situation. Again the person may need support from the leader at this point, but remember it is OK for people with dementia to show and talk about emotions in the group, if they wish to.

What if some members are really reluctant or are not enjoying the sessions?

Think carefully about what is leading some members to not enjoy the sessions. Is it being run at too high a level for them – are

they finding it too challenging? Or, is it the other way round? Perhaps they are bored with the group, as it is all too easy for them. Look at ways of adapting the sessions so that there is more for these members to enjoy and feel positive about. Perhaps there is friction between certain group members or some are highly critical of others. Group leaders need to ensure that vulnerable members of the group are protected, and through ensuring they experience success in the group, help to boost their self-esteem. Sometimes people seem reluctant to come to the group, but enjoy it when they get there. It's quite possible that, sitting in a comfortable seat in the day room, being asked to go to a meeting which they cannot remember ever hearing about before, inertia sets in. Only when in the room, with the fellow members, the warm, positive memories of the group surface again. Where the person refuses to attend, despite efforts to prompt and remind, this decision must, of course, be respected.

What if no one in the group wants to sing?

Having established members' likes and dislikes, use a tape to bring members' favourite music into the group, and encourage members to move to the music or use simple percussion instruments to accompany it. Before too long members will be singing along to the tape, if it has been well chosen.

What if we can't get all the equipment?

Improvise! The programme is not intended to be rigid, but to give ideas and to stimulate your own creativity, ideas and thinking. Good luck!

Further reading

Orrell M, Spector A, Thorgrimsen L, Woods R (2005) A pilot study examining the effectiveness of maintenance cognitive stimulation therapy (CST) following CST for people with dementia. *International Journal of Geriatric Psychiatry* 20 446-451.

Spector A, Thorgrimsen L, Woods B, Royan L, Davies S, Butterworth M, Orrell M (2003) Efficacy of an evidence-based cognitive stimulation therapy programme for people with dementia: randomised controlled trial. *British Journal of Psychiatry* 183 248-254.

Spector A, Orrell M, Davies S, Woods B (2001) Can Reality Orientation be rehabilitated? Development and piloting of an evidence-based programme of cognition-based therapies for people with dementia. *Neuropsychological Rehabilitation* 11(3/4) 377-397.

Spector A, Davies S, Woods B, Orrell M (2000) Reality orientation for dementia: a systematic review of the evidence for its effectiveness. *Gerontologist* 40 206-212.

Holden UP, Woods RT (1995). *Positive approaches to dementia care* (3rd edition). Churchill Livingstone, Edinburgh.